HYPERBARIC OXYGEN HEALING ADVANTAGE

Exploring the healing depths
of Hyperbaric Oxygen
Therapy to revolutionise and
hasten recovery from
various health conditions

Dr Andy Brighton

Table Of Contents

OVERVIEW

Definition and History of Hyperbaric Oxygen Therapy (HBOT)

Hyperbaric Oxygen Therapy (HBOT) involves breathing pure oxygen in a pressurized room or chamber. The increased pressure allows the lungs to gather more oxygen than normal, enhancing the body's natural healing processes. This therapy has diverse applications, ranging from treating chronic wounds to addressing neurological conditions.

The history of HBOT can be traced back to the 17th century when English physician Henshaw built a sealed chamber to explore the effects of increased atmospheric pressure. However, it wasn't until the 20th century that HBOT gained medical significance. The treatment found its footing during World War I and World War II for treating decompression sickness in divers.

The modern era has seen an expansion of HBOT applications, with ongoing research uncovering new therapeutic possibilities. Today, it stands as a crucial element in the medical field, continually evolving as researchers delve deeper into its mechanisms and potential benefits.

The book aims to provide a comprehensive understanding of hyperbaric oxygen therapy, offering a blend of scientific insights and practical information. It is structured to guide both healthcare professionals and the general audience through the intricate landscape of HBOT.

Readers will embark on a journey from the basics, exploring the fundamental concepts of HBOT, to the advanced applications across various medical conditions. The book is not only an informative resource but also a practical guide for those considering or undergoing hyperbaric oxygen therapy.

Each chapter delves into different facets of HBOT, starting with its mechanisms and physiological effects. The diverse types of hyperbaric chambers are discussed, shedding light on the technology driving this therapeutic approach. The book then navigates through specific conditions treated with HBOT, including wound healing, decompression sickness, and the emerging applications in neurological disorders and pediatrics.

The narrative includes real-life stories and testimonials, offering a human touch to the scientific exploration. Safety considerations and potential side effects are addressed to ensure a balanced understanding, empowering readers with knowledge for informed decision-making.

Furthermore, the book explores the current research landscape, highlighting ongoing studies and potential future directions. Safety protocols, collaboration with healthcare professionals, and the integration of HBOT into clinical practice are emphasized, providing practical insights for medical professionals interested in incorporating this therapy into their toolkit.

In the concluding chapters, the book offers a reflection on the future of hyperbaric oxygen therapy, envisioning potential innovations and areas for further research. A comprehensive glossary, resources for additional reading, and an index enhance the book's utility as a reference guide.

In essence, this book serves as a beacon, illuminating the depths of hyperbaric oxygen therapy, from its historical roots to the forefront of medical advancements. Whether you're a healthcare professional, a patient, or someone curious about the healing potential of oxygen, this book endeavors to be a valuable companion in your exploration of hyperbaric oxygen therapy.

CHAPTER ONE

Understanding Hyperbaric Oxygen Therapy

Mechanism of Action

The effectiveness of Hyperbaric Oxygen Therapy (HBOT) lies in its intricate mechanism of action, which harnesses the healing power of oxygen under increased atmospheric pressure. When a person undergoes HBOT, they breathe pure oxygen within a sealed chamber, where the pressure is higher than atmospheric pressure.

At elevated pressures, oxygen dissolves into the bloodstream at significantly higher concentrations. This hyperoxygenation serves two primary purposes. First, it enhances the oxygen-carrying capacity of red blood cells, ensuring more efficient oxygen delivery to tissues. Second, it allows oxygen to dissolve directly into plasma, reaching areas with compromised blood flow, such as damaged tissues or wounds.

Additionally, HBOT triggers the release of growth factors and stem cells, promoting tissue regeneration. The therapy also has anti-inflammatory effects by modulating immune responses, reducing oxidative stress, and decreasing the expression of inflammatory markers.

Understanding the molecular and cellular changes induced by HBOT provides insight into its versatility. From aiding in wound healing to mitigating the impact of neurological injuries, the therapy's mechanism adapts to different physiological contexts.

Physiological Effects on the Body

HBOT exerts a profound impact on various physiological processes, influencing both systemic and localized responses within the body. One of the primary effects is increased oxygen delivery to tissues. This enhanced oxygenation contributes to improved cellular metabolism, facilitating energy production and supporting the body's natural healing mechanisms.

The therapy is particularly beneficial for wound healing. Elevated oxygen levels enhance collagen formation, accelerate tissue repair, and promote the formation of new blood vessels (angiogenesis). This makes HBOT an effective adjunctive treatment for chronic wounds, non-healing ulcers, and tissue damage caused by radiation therapy.

In neurological applications, HBOT demonstrates neuroprotective effects. It has been studied for conditions such as stroke and traumatic brain injury, where the increased oxygen availability helps mitigate secondary damage, reduce inflammation, and support neuronal recovery. The therapy's influence extends to neuroplasticity, enhancing the brain's ability to adapt and repair.

HBOT also plays a role in combating infections. Oxygen is a potent antimicrobial agent, and the increased levels delivered during therapy create an inhospitable environment for certain bacteria and fungi. This antimicrobial effect contributes to the management of infections, particularly in cases of chronic osteomyelitis or compromised wound healing.

However, it's essential to note that the physiological effects of HBOT are context-dependent. While it offers benefits in specific conditions, its application is not universally suitable. Understanding the nuanced interactions between elevated oxygen levels and different bodily systems is crucial for optimizing therapeutic outcomes.

Indications and Contraindications

HBOT has a diverse range of indications, making it a versatile therapeutic modality. Understanding when to consider HBOT involves recognizing conditions where enhanced oxygenation can positively impact outcomes.

Indications

1. Wound Healing: Chronic wounds, diabetic foot ulcers, and non-healing surgical wounds benefit from HBOT's ability to stimulate tissue repair and angiogenesis.

2. Decompression Sickness:

Commonly known as "the bends," this condition occurs in divers ascending too quickly. HBOT helps eliminate nitrogen bubbles in the bloodstream.

3. Carbon Monoxide Poisoning: By accelerating the elimination of carbon monoxide from the body and promoting tissue oxygenation, HBOT is a crucial intervention in cases of poisoning.

4. Radiation Injury: HBOT aids in the recovery of tissues damaged by radiation therapy, reducing side effects and promoting healing.

Contraindications:

1.   Untreated   Pneumothorax: The
increased   pressure   during   HBOT   can
exacerbate   an   untreated   pneumothorax,
where   air   leaks   into   the   space   between
the lungs and chest wall.

2.   Certain   Respiratory   Conditions:
Individuals   with   chronic   obstructive
pulmonary   disease   (COPD)   or   severe
respiratory   infections   may   face
challenges in tolerating increased oxygen
levels.

3. Claustrophobia: The enclosed nature
of   hyperbaric   chambers   may   be

unsuitable for individuals with severe claustrophobia.

4. Seizure Disorders: While the relationship between HBOT and seizures is complex, caution is exercised in individuals with uncontrolled seizure disorders.

5. Pregnancy: Limited data are available on the safety of HBOT during pregnancy, and caution is exercised to avoid potential risks to the fetus.

Understanding the nuanced interplay of these indications and contraindications is vital for healthcare professionals prescribing HBOT and patients considering or undergoing the therapy. A thoughtful evaluation of the individual's medical history, the nature of the condition, and the potential benefits and risks guides the decision-making process, ensuring that HBOT is employed judiciously for optimal outcomes.

CHAPTER TWO

Types of Hyperbaric Chambers

Monoplace Chambers:

Monoplace hyperbaric chambers are designed to accommodate a single person during a treatment session. These chambers are typically transparent or have clear viewing ports, helping alleviate feelings of claustrophobia. The patient lies on a treatment table that slides into the chamber, and once inside, the chamber is pressurized with 100% oxygen.

One of the primary advantages of monoplace chambers is their simplicity and ease of operation. The focused environment allows for personalized treatment plans tailored to individual patient needs. Additionally, the transparency of the chamber helps medical staff monitor and communicate with the patient throughout the session, enhancing the overall experience.

Monoplace chambers are often used in hospital settings, outpatient facilities, or private clinics. Their compact design and efficiency make them suitable for a wide range of applications, including wound healing, carbon monoxide poisoning, and certain neurological conditions. However, due to their single-patient capacity, they may not be the most time-efficient option for larger healthcare facilities with high patient volumes.

Multiplace Chambers:

In contrast to monoplace chambers, multiplace hyperbaric chambers are designed to accommodate multiple individuals simultaneously. These chambers are pressurized with air, and patients breathe pure oxygen through masks or hoods during the treatment. The chamber's large size allows medical staff, such as nurses and technicians, to be present inside during the session, providing direct patient care and monitoring.

Multiplace chambers offer advantages in terms of efficiency, as they can treat multiple patients concurrently, making them suitable for hospitals or large healthcare facilities with a high patient throughput. The ability to provide care directly within the chamber ensures immediate response to any issues that may arise during treatment. The larger space also allows for certain medical interventions to be performed, enhancing the versatility of the chamber.

However, the use of air as the pressurizing gas in multiplace chambers requires patients to breathe oxygen through masks or hoods, which can be less comfortable than breathing 100% oxygen in a monoplace chamber. Despite this, multiplace chambers remain a practical and effective solution for a variety of conditions, including decompression sickness and chronic non-healing wounds.

Portable Chambers:

Portable hyperbaric chambers, also known as mild hyperbaric chambers, are a more recent development in the field of hyperbaric oxygen therapy. Unlike monoplace and multiplace chambers, portable chambers are typically soft-sided and can be transported and set up in various locations. These chambers are pressurized with ambient air, and patients breathe concentrated oxygen through a mask.

The portability of these chambers offers flexibility in terms of treatment location, making them suitable for outpatient clinics, wellness centers, or even in-home use. However, it's important to note that portable chambers operate at lower pressures compared to traditional chambers, which can impact the level of oxygen dissolved in the bloodstream.

Portable chambers are considered for conditions where mild hyperbaric therapy is sufficient, such as general wellness, fatigue, or certain neurological conditions. They are not typically used for critical medical conditions that require the higher pressures provided by monoplace or multiplace chambers.

Considerations in Choosing a Hyperbaric Chamber:

Selecting the appropriate type of hyperbaric chamber depends on various factors, including the nature of the medical condition being treated, the available space in the healthcare facility, patient comfort, and the desired treatment protocol.

1. Medical Condition: Different chambers may be more suitable for specific medical conditions. Monoplace chambers, with their focused treatment environment, are often preferred for wound healing, while multiplace chambers are efficient for conditions like decompression sickness.

2. Space and Throughput: The size and capacity of the facility play a role in choosing between monoplace and

multiplace chambers. Hospitals with high patient volumes may benefit from the efficiency of multiplace chambers, while smaller clinics or those with space constraints may find monoplace chambers more practical.

3. Patient Comfort and Preferences: Some patients may have a preference for the transparency of monoplace chambers, which can help alleviate feelings of claustrophobia. Others may appreciate the social aspect of multiplace chambers, where they can undergo treatment alongside family or friends.

4. Treatment Protocol: The prescribed treatment protocol, including pressure and duration, may influence the choice of chamber. Conditions requiring higher pressures or specialized medical interventions may necessitate the use of multiplace chambers.

5. Portability and Convenience: Portable chambers offer the advantage of mobility, making them suitable for locations where traditional chambers may not be feasible. However, their lower pressure capabilities limit their use for certain medical conditions.

In conclusion, the choice between monoplace, multiplace, or portable hyperbaric chambers involves careful consideration of various factors. Each type has its unique advantages and applications, contributing to the versatility of hyperbaric oxygen therapy across different healthcare settings. As technology advances, ongoing research and innovation in chamber design continue to shape the landscape of hyperbaric medicine, expanding its accessibility and effectiveness in diverse medical contexts.

CHAPTER THREE

Conditions Treated with Hyperbaric Oxygen Therapy (HBOT)

Wound Healing:

Hyperbaric Oxygen Therapy (HBOT) has demonstrated remarkable efficacy in promoting wound healing, especially in cases where conventional treatments have proven inadequate. The therapy's ability to enhance oxygen delivery to tissues plays a pivotal role in various stages of wound repair.

In chronic wounds, such as diabetic foot ulcers or non-healing surgical wounds, inadequate oxygen supply can impede the normal healing process. HBOT addresses this challenge by saturating the bloodstream with increased levels of oxygen. This, in turn, stimulates angiogenesis (the formation of new blood vessels) and collagen synthesis, crucial components of tissue regeneration.

The hyperoxygenation facilitated by HBOT also bolsters the activity of white blood cells, promoting an antimicrobial environment. This is particularly beneficial in cases where infections complicate the wound healing process.

By enhancing the body's natural defenses, HBOT contributes to the resolution of infections and accelerates the overall healing trajectory.

Moreover, HBOT is utilized in cases of crush injuries or traumatic wounds where compromised blood supply poses a significant challenge. The therapy aids in salvaging damaged tissues by providing the necessary oxygen levels to support cellular metabolism and minimize secondary damage.

Decompression Sickness:

Decompression sickness (DCS), commonly known as "the bends," is a condition that can occur when divers ascend too quickly, leading to the formation of nitrogen bubbles in the bloodstream. HBOT is a primary and highly effective treatment for DCS, providing a means to eliminate these nitrogen bubbles and alleviate symptoms.

During a dive, the body absorbs increased amounts of nitrogen due to the elevated pressure underwater. If a diver ascends too rapidly, the reduced pressure allows nitrogen to form bubbles, leading to symptoms such as joint pain, dizziness, and, in severe cases, neurological complications. HBOT addresses DCS by recompressing the diver in a hyperbaric chamber, effectively reducing the size of the nitrogen bubbles and promoting their elimination.

The pressurized environment in the hyperbaric chamber facilitates the dissolution of nitrogen back into the bloodstream, allowing the body to safely expel it through respiration. Timely administration of HBOT is crucial in DCS cases to prevent the progression of symptoms and minimize potential long-term complications.

Carbon Monoxide Poisoning:

Carbon monoxide (CO) poisoning occurs when individuals are exposed to high levels of carbon monoxide gas, often from incomplete combustion of fuels. CO binds strongly to hemoglobin, reducing the blood's oxygen-carrying capacity and leading to hypoxia. HBOT is a critical intervention in cases of severe carbon monoxide poisoning.

In a hyperbaric chamber, the increased atmospheric pressure accelerates the elimination of carbon monoxide from the body. Breathing 100% oxygen in this pressurized environment enhances the displacement of CO from hemoglobin and promotes its elimination through the lungs. This process is significantly faster than breathing ambient air at normal atmospheric pressure.

HBOT not only helps in removing carbon monoxide but also mitigates the long-term neurological effects associated with severe poisoning. By improving oxygen delivery to tissues, particularly the brain, it supports the recovery of neural function and reduces the risk of cognitive and neurological sequelae.

Radiation Injury:

Patients undergoing radiation therapy for cancer may experience side effects that impact surrounding tissues, leading to conditions known as radiation injury or radiation-induced tissue damage. HBOT has emerged as a valuable adjunctive therapy for managing and mitigating the effects of radiation injury.

Radiation can cause damage to blood vessels and connective tissues, impairing normal wound healing processes. HBOT addresses these challenges by promoting angiogenesis and enhancing tissue oxygenation. The therapy facilitates the recovery of damaged tissues, reducing inflammation, promoting collagen formation, and supporting the overall healing response.

In cases of osteoradionecrosis, a condition where radiation therapy affects the bone, HBOT has been shown to be effective in promoting bone healing and preventing further deterioration. By stimulating the formation of new blood vessels and supporting cellular metabolism, HBOT contributes to the restoration of bone health in affected areas.

Moreover, HBOT is considered in cases of soft tissue radiation injury, where the therapy aids in reducing fibrosis and improving the elasticity of affected tissues. This multifaceted approach makes HBOT a valuable component of comprehensive care for individuals dealing with the aftermath of radiation therapy.

In conclusion, Hyperbaric Oxygen Therapy demonstrates its versatility in addressing a range of medical conditions, from wound healing complications to the intricate challenges posed by decompression sickness, carbon monoxide poisoning, and radiation injury. The therapy's ability to harness the healing potential of oxygen under increased atmospheric pressure has positioned it as an essential modality in modern medicine, offering hope and healing across diverse clinical scenarios.

CHAPTER FOUR

Application in Neurological Disorders

Stroke:

Hyperbaric Oxygen Therapy (HBOT) has emerged as a promising adjunctive treatment for individuals who have experienced a stroke, a condition where a disruption of blood flow to the brain results in damage to brain cells. The therapeutic application of HBOT in stroke revolves around its ability to address two critical aspects: reducing inflammation and promoting neuroplasticity.

During a stroke, the affected brain tissue often experiences reduced oxygen supply, leading to inflammation and the formation of reactive oxygen species. HBOT helps mitigate this inflammatory response by delivering high levels of oxygen to the affected area. The increased oxygen availability supports cellular metabolism, reduces oxidative stress, and contributes to the resolution of inflammation.

Furthermore, HBOT plays a role in neuroplasticity, the brain's ability to reorganize itself by forming new neural connections. Post-stroke, the brain undergoes a complex process of rewiring to compensate for the damaged areas. The oxygen-rich environment created by HBOT supports these neuroplastic changes, potentially enhancing the recovery of motor function and cognitive abilities.

Research studies and clinical trials exploring the impact of HBOT on stroke recovery have shown promising results. While the therapy is not a standalone treatment for stroke, it is considered a valuable complement to conventional rehabilitation strategies, offering the potential to accelerate recovery and improve overall outcomes.

Traumatic Brain Injury:

Traumatic Brain Injury (TBI) poses significant challenges due to the complex and often unpredictable nature of the injury. HBOT has garnered attention as a potential therapeutic intervention for TBI, with its mechanisms of action aiming to address various aspects of the injury's pathophysiology.

In cases of TBI, the initial trauma triggers a cascade of events, including inflammation, reduced blood flow, and the release of neurotoxic substances. HBOT addresses these processes by promoting oxygen delivery to the injured brain tissue. The therapy helps counteract hypoxia (low oxygen levels), supports cellular metabolism, and contributes to the resolution of inflammation.

Additionally, HBOT has been shown to have neuroprotective effects, reducing secondary damage that may occur in the hours and days following the initial injury. The therapy's impact on mitigating oxidative stress and supporting the brain's natural repair mechanisms contributes to its potential in TBI management.

Clinical studies exploring the use of HBOT in TBI have demonstrated mixed results, and the optimal protocols for treatment are still a subject of ongoing research. However, the potential benefits observed in some cases, such as improved cognitive function and reduced long-term complications, highlight the need for further exploration of HBOT's role in the comprehensive care of individuals with traumatic brain injuries.

Neurodegenerative Diseases:

The application of Hyperbaric Oxygen Therapy in neurodegenerative diseases represents a growing area of interest within the medical community. While not a cure, HBOT holds promise in managing symptoms and potentially influencing the progression of certain neurodegenerative conditions, including Alzheimer's disease, Parkinson's disease, and amyotrophic lateral sclerosis (ALS).

In Alzheimer's disease, characterized by the accumulation of beta-amyloid plaques in the brain, HBOT's potential lies in its ability to improve oxygenation and support cognitive function. The therapy's anti-inflammatory effects may also contribute to the reduction of neuroinflammation associated with Alzheimer's.

Parkinson's disease involves the degeneration of dopamine-producing neurons in the brain. While the exact mechanisms are still under investigation, some studies suggest that HBOT may have neuroprotective effects, potentially slowing the progression of the disease. The therapy's impact on mitochondrial function and cellular metabolism is of particular interest in the context of neurodegenerative disorders.

In ALS, a progressive motor neuron disease, the potential benefits of HBOT are being explored in preclinical and clinical settings. The therapy's ability to enhance oxygen delivery to tissues and mitigate inflammation may have implications for the preservation of motor function in individuals with ALS.

While research in this area is still in its early stages, the multifaceted mechanisms of action of HBOT make it a compelling avenue for exploration in the realm of neurodegenerative diseases. It's important to note that individual responses to HBOT may vary, and the therapy is not a substitute for established treatments. Ongoing research aims to refine protocols, identify specific subpopulations that may benefit most, and further elucidate the underlying mechanisms that make HBOT a potentially valuable component in the management of neurodegenerative conditions.

In summary, Hyperbaric Oxygen Therapy demonstrates promise in the realm of neurological disorders, offering a multifaceted approach to addressing the complexities of stroke, traumatic brain injury, and neurodegenerative diseases. While the field continues to evolve with ongoing research, the potential for HBOT to complement existing treatments and improve outcomes for individuals dealing with these challenging conditions underscores its significance in the landscape of modern neurotherapeutics.

CHAPTER FIVE

Pediatric Applications

Cerebral Palsy:

Hyperbaric Oxygen Therapy (HBOT) has gained attention for its potential applications in pediatric neurology, particularly in the management of conditions like Cerebral Palsy (CP). CP is a group of neurological disorders affecting movement and posture, often stemming from damage to the developing brain during pregnancy, childbirth, or early infancy.

HBOT's role in CP is rooted in its ability to enhance oxygen delivery to tissues, potentially mitigating the effects of hypoxia and promoting neuroplasticity. In the context of CP, where impaired motor function is a primary concern, the therapy aims to address both the underlying neurological factors and associated complications.

The increased oxygen levels provided by HBOT contribute to improved cellular metabolism and support the brain's natural repair mechanisms. Studies exploring the use of HBOT in CP have reported positive outcomes, including enhanced motor function, reduced spasticity, and improvements in activities of daily living.

The therapy's impact on inflammation is also noteworthy, as neuroinflammation is implicated in the progression of CP. By modulating immune responses and reducing oxidative stress, HBOT may help create a more favorable environment for neurological recovery.

It's essential to note that the application of HBOT in pediatric cases, including CP, requires careful consideration of individualized treatment plans. The age, severity of symptoms, and specific challenges faced by each child influence the decision to incorporate HBOT into the overall management approach. Collaborative efforts between healthcare professionals, including pediatric neurologists and rehabilitation specialists, play a crucial role in determining the appropriateness and potential benefits of HBOT for children with CP.

Autism Spectrum Disorders:

The exploration of Hyperbaric Oxygen Therapy (HBOT) in the realm of pediatric neurology extends to Autism Spectrum Disorders (ASD). ASD encompasses a range of neurodevelopmental conditions characterized by challenges in social interaction, communication, and repetitive behaviors. While the causes of ASD are complex and multifactorial, research has explored the potential benefits of HBOT as a complementary intervention.

In ASD, abnormalities in brain structure, function, and connectivity have been identified. HBOT's mechanisms of action, including enhanced oxygen delivery and anti-inflammatory effects, are hypothesized to influence these neurological aspects. By providing increased levels of oxygen to brain tissues, the therapy aims to support cellular metabolism, reduce oxidative stress, and potentially modulate neuroinflammation.

While the body of evidence exploring HBOT in ASD is growing, it's important to approach the topic with a nuanced perspective. Research outcomes vary, and the optimal protocols for treatment are still under investigation. Some studies have reported improvements in certain behaviors, communication skills, and social interactions in individuals with ASD following HBOT. However, challenges such as the heterogeneity of ASD and the need for larger, well-controlled studies contribute to the ongoing discourse on the therapy's efficacy in this context.

The decision to consider HBOT in pediatric cases of ASD requires a comprehensive evaluation by healthcare professionals, including pediatric neurologists, developmental pediatricians, and other specialists. Individualized treatment plans, consideration of the child's age, and collaboration with families are crucial aspects of navigating the potential role of HBOT in the management of ASD.

Considerations in Pediatric Applications:

When exploring the application of Hyperbaric Oxygen Therapy (HBOT) in pediatric cases, several considerations come into play to ensure the safety and appropriateness of the therapy for young patients.

1. Age and Developmental Stage: The age of the child and their developmental stage influence the potential benefits and risks of HBOT. Pediatric patients may require specialized approaches to make

the experience more comfortable and less anxiety-inducing.

2.   Collaboration with Pediatric Specialists: Successful integration of HBOT into pediatric care involves collaboration with a multidisciplinary team of healthcare professionals. Pediatric neurologists, developmental pediatricians, rehabilitation specialists, and other experts contribute their insights to create comprehensive treatment plans.

3. Individualized Treatment Plans: Children with neurological conditions often present with unique challenges and

diverse needs. Individualized treatment plans consider the specific characteristics of the child's condition, the severity of symptoms, and the family's preferences and expectations.

4. Monitoring and Assessment: Regular monitoring and assessment are crucial components of pediatric HBOT applications. Objective measures, such as neuroimaging and standardized assessments, help track progress and guide adjustments to the treatment plan.

5. Informed Consent and Family Involvement: Informed consent from parents or guardians is a fundamental

aspect of pediatric HBOT applications. Open communication with families, addressing their questions and concerns, and involving them in decision-making contribute to a collaborative and supportive care environment.

6. Safety Protocols: Safety protocols specific to pediatric cases are essential to ensure the well-being of young patients. Proper training of medical staff, adherence to established guidelines, and continuous monitoring during HBOT sessions contribute to a safe therapeutic experience.

7. Ethical Considerations: Ethical considerations play a significant role in pediatric healthcare decisions. Transparent communication with families, respect for autonomy, and adherence to ethical standards guide the ethical application of HBOT in pediatric cases.

In conclusion, the exploration of Hyperbaric Oxygen Therapy in pediatric neurology reflects a dynamic and evolving field. From addressing the challenges of Cerebral Palsy to investigating the potential benefits in Autism Spectrum Disorders, the application of HBOT in pediatric cases requires a nuanced and collaborative approach. Ongoing research, multidisciplinary collaboration, and a commitment to individualized care contribute to the continued exploration of HBOT's role in supporting the neurological well-being of children.

CHAPTER SIX

Research and Advances in HBOT

Ongoing Studies:

The landscape of Hyperbaric Oxygen Therapy (HBOT) is continuously evolving, with ongoing research studies exploring its efficacy, mechanisms of action, and potential applications across diverse medical conditions. These studies contribute to the refinement of treatment protocols, the identification of optimal patient populations, and the expansion of HBOT into new realms of healthcare.

1. Traumatic Brain Injury (TBI): Ongoing research delves into the impact of HBOT on Traumatic Brain Injury, with a focus on elucidating the specific mechanisms that contribute to neuroprotection and recovery. Studies aim to determine the most effective treatment protocols, including pressure levels and session durations, to maximize positive outcomes for individuals with TBI.

2. Chronic Wounds: The application of HBOT in chronic wound healing remains a robust area of investigation. Studies explore its effectiveness in various wound types, including diabetic ulcers, non-healing surgical wounds, and

pressure sores. Researchers aim to refine protocols to optimize healing rates, reduce complications, and enhance the overall quality of life for patients with chronic wounds.

3. Neurological Disorders: Ongoing studies in the realm of neurology continue to explore the potential of HBOT in conditions such as stroke, Alzheimer's disease, and Parkinson's disease. Researchers investigate the therapy's impact on neuroplasticity, neuroinflammation, and cognitive function, contributing to the understanding of how HBOT can be

integrated into comprehensive treatment approaches for neurological disorders.

4. Post-Concussion Syndrome: The role of HBOT in addressing symptoms of Post-Concussion Syndrome is a subject of ongoing research. Studies aim to determine whether the therapy can provide relief from persistent symptoms such as headaches, cognitive impairment, and emotional disturbances in individuals who have experienced concussions.

5. Inflammatory Bowel Disease (IBD): Emerging research explores the potential benefits of HBOT in Inflammatory Bowel

Disease, including conditions like Crohn's disease and ulcerative colitis. The anti-inflammatory effects of HBOT are of particular interest in mitigating the inflammatory processes associated with IBD and promoting tissue healing.

6. Cancer Treatment Support: Ongoing studies investigate the role of HBOT as a supportive therapy in cancer treatment. Researchers explore whether HBOT can enhance the effectiveness of certain cancer treatments, reduce side effects, and improve the overall well-being of individuals undergoing cancer therapy.

7. Psychiatric Conditions: Some studies explore the impact of HBOT on psychiatric conditions, including depression and post-traumatic stress disorder (PTSD). Researchers investigate whether the therapy's influence on neuroplasticity and neurotransmitter function may have positive effects on mood and emotional well-being.

8. Aging and Cognitive Decline: The potential of HBOT in addressing age-related cognitive decline and promoting cognitive resilience is a growing area of interest. Studies aim to uncover the neuroprotective mechanisms

of HBOT and its impact on cognitive function in aging populations.

These ongoing studies represent just a snapshot of the dynamic research landscape surrounding HBOT. Collaborative efforts from researchers, clinicians, and healthcare institutions worldwide contribute to the accumulation of knowledge that shapes the future of hyperbaric medicine.

Emerging Therapeutic Areas:

Beyond ongoing studies, Hyperbaric Oxygen Therapy is exploring emerging therapeutic areas, pushing the boundaries of its applications and uncovering new possibilities for improving patient outcomes. These emerging areas showcase the versatility of HBOT and its potential impact on diverse aspects of health and well-being.

1. Regenerative Medicine: HBOT's ability to stimulate stem cell activity and promote tissue regeneration aligns with the goals of regenerative medicine. Researchers are exploring how HBOT can be integrated into regenerative approaches for conditions involving tissue damage, injury, or degeneration.

2. Dermatology: Emerging research in dermatology explores the potential of HBOT in addressing skin conditions, such as wound healing after dermatological procedures, reducing inflammation in inflammatory skin disorders, and supporting the recovery of damaged skin.

3. Sports Medicine: Athletes and sports medicine professionals are exploring the role of HBOT in sports-related injuries and recovery. Studies investigate its potential in accelerating the healing of musculoskeletal injuries, reducing inflammation, and enhancing overall recovery for athletes.

4. Metabolic Disorders: The impact of HBOT on metabolic disorders, including conditions like diabetes, is an area of increasing interest. Researchers explore how the therapy may contribute to improved wound healing, reduced complications associated with diabetes, and enhanced vascular health.

5. Preventive Medicine: Some research initiatives explore the potential of HBOT as a preventive measure, particularly in aging populations. Investigations focus on whether regular HBOT sessions can contribute to cognitive resilience, reduce

the risk of certain age-related conditions, and promote overall well-being.

6. Combination Therapies: Researchers are exploring the synergies between HBOT and other therapeutic modalities. This includes investigating how combining HBOT with traditional medical treatments, physical therapy, or complementary therapies may enhance overall treatment outcomes for various conditions.

7. Vascular Health: The impact of HBOT on vascular health, including its potential role in improving blood vessel function and reducing the risk of cardiovascular

complications, is an emerging area of investigation. Studies aim to uncover how HBOT may positively influence vascular health beyond its immediate applications.

8. Dental and Oral Health: Emerging research explores the applications of HBOT in dentistry, including its potential role in supporting the healing of oral tissues after procedures, reducing inflammation in periodontal conditions, and promoting overall oral health.

As the field of hyperbaric medicine continues to advance, the exploration of emerging therapeutic areas reflects the commitment of researchers and healthcare professionals to uncover the full spectrum of possibilities offered by HBOT. These emerging frontiers hold the promise of expanding the therapeutic reach of HBOT and contributing to innovative approaches in healthcare.

In conclusion, the dynamic landscape of research and advances in Hyperbaric Oxygen Therapy highlights its versatility and potential impact across a spectrum of medical conditions. Ongoing studies and emerging therapeutic areas contribute to the evolving understanding of HBOT, shaping its role in modern medicine and paving the way for innovative applications that enhance patient care and well-being.

CHAPTER SEVEN

Safety and Side Effects

Safety Protocols:

Hyperbaric Oxygen Therapy (HBOT) is generally considered safe when administered by trained healthcare professionals in controlled environments. However, adherence to safety protocols is crucial to mitigate potential risks and ensure the well-being of patients undergoing HBOT sessions.

1. Qualified Personnel: HBOT should be administered by qualified and

experienced healthcare professionals, including hyperbaric medicine physicians, certified hyperbaric nurses, and technicians trained in chamber operations. Their expertise ensures proper supervision, response to emergencies, and adherence to established safety guidelines.

2. Chamber Integrity: Regular maintenance and inspection of hyperbaric chambers are essential to ensure their integrity. Chambers must meet safety standards, and any issues with seals, valves, or pressure systems must be promptly addressed to prevent leaks or malfunctions.

3. Fire Safety Measures: Given the enriched oxygen environment within hyperbaric chambers, fire safety measures are paramount. Non-flammable materials should be used in chamber construction, and strict protocols for preventing and responding to fires must be in place.

4. Patient Monitoring: Continuous monitoring of patients during HBOT sessions is crucial. Vital signs, oxygen saturation levels, and patient comfort are closely observed. Monitoring systems inside the chamber facilitate real-time

communication between healthcare professionals and patients.

5. Emergency Procedures: Well-defined emergency procedures should be in place, including protocols for rapid decompression, fire emergencies, and evacuation. Healthcare providers undergo training to respond effectively to various emergency scenarios that may arise during HBOT sessions.

6. Patient Education: Informing patients about the procedures, potential side effects, and safety measures is an integral part of HBOT. Patients receive pre-session briefings, and any concerns

or questions are addressed to ensure they have a clear understanding of what to expect.

7. Compliance with Guidelines: Adherence to established guidelines and standards, such as those set by medical organizations and regulatory bodies, is fundamental. Healthcare facilities offering HBOT must comply with safety and operational protocols to maintain a high standard of care.

By implementing rigorous safety protocols, healthcare providers can create a secure environment for the administration of HBOT, minimizing the risks associated with this therapeutic modality.

Common Side Effects:

While Hyperbaric Oxygen Therapy (HBOT) is generally safe, patients may experience certain side effects, most of which are mild and transient. Understanding these side effects is essential for both healthcare providers and patients.

1. Barotrauma: Changes in pressure during the compression and decompression phases of HBOT can lead to barotrauma, affecting the ears,

sinuses, and teeth. Patients are instructed on techniques, such as equalizing ear pressure, to minimize the risk of barotrauma.

2. Oxygen Toxicity: Prolonged exposure to high levels of oxygen can lead to oxygen toxicity, which may manifest as seizures. To mitigate this risk, healthcare providers carefully monitor oxygen levels, session durations, and individual patient tolerance. Seizures are a rare but serious side effect that requires prompt intervention.

3. Claustrophobia: The enclosed nature of hyperbaric chambers may trigger

feelings of claustrophobia in some patients. Pre-session education, psychological support, and the option for shorter introductory sessions can help manage this side effect.

4. Temporary Vision Changes: Some patients may experience temporary changes in vision, such as nearsightedness or farsightedness. These changes typically resolve after completing the HBOT sessions.

5. Fatigue: Mild fatigue is a common side effect, especially after the initial sessions. Patients are advised to rest and allow their bodies to adjust to the therapy.

6. Sinus or Ear Discomfort: Changes in pressure can lead to discomfort in the sinuses or ears. Proper equalization techniques, such as swallowing or yawning, can alleviate these sensations.

It's crucial to note that the majority of side effects associated with HBOT are short-lived and resolve once the sessions are completed. Healthcare providers carefully monitor patients during sessions to address any emerging issues promptly.

Patient Screening:

Patient screening is a critical component of the safety protocols associated with Hyperbaric Oxygen Therapy (HBOT). Thorough screening helps identify individuals who may have contraindications or conditions that require special consideration before undergoing HBOT.

1. Medical History Review: A comprehensive review of the patient's medical history is conducted to identify any pre-existing conditions, surgeries, or

medications that may influence the suitability of HBOT.

2. Contraindications: Certain medical conditions may contraindicate HBOT. For example, untreated pneumothorax, severe respiratory conditions, and specific medications may pose challenges during hyperbaric sessions. Patients with these contraindications may not be suitable candidates for HBOT.

3. Assessment of Oxygen Tolerance: Individuals with a history of seizures or conditions that may increase susceptibility to oxygen toxicity are carefully evaluated. This assessment

helps determine the appropriate oxygen levels and session durations to minimize the risk of seizures.

4. Evaluation of Claustrophobia Risk: Patients with a history of claustrophobia or anxiety disorders may be at an increased risk of experiencing psychological discomfort during HBOT. Open communication, education, and gradual acclimatization may be employed to address these concerns.

5. Pregnancy Screening: Limited data are available regarding the safety of HBOT during pregnancy, and caution is exercised. Pregnancy screening is crucial,

and the potential risks and benefits are carefully considered before recommending HBOT for pregnant individuals.

6. Communication with Patients: Open communication with patients is key to ensuring their comfort and understanding of the screening process. Patients are encouraged to disclose any relevant information about their health, and any questions or concerns are addressed by healthcare providers.

7. Informed Consent: Informed consent is an integral part of the screening process. Patients receive detailed

information about the procedures, potential risks, and expected outcomes of HBOT. This ensures that patients make informed decisions and actively participate in their healthcare.

By conducting thorough patient screening, healthcare providers can identify individuals who are suitable candidates for HBOT and tailor the therapy to individual needs, minimizing risks and optimizing the potential benefits.

In conclusion, the safety and side effects of Hyperbaric Oxygen Therapy are carefully managed through robust safety protocols, thorough patient screening, and continuous monitoring during sessions. By prioritizing patient safety, healthcare providers ensure that HBOT remains a valuable and well-tolerated therapeutic modality across a diverse range

CHAPTER EIGHT

Patient Stories and Testimonials

The journey of healing often extends beyond the realms of clinical studies and medical literature. Personal narratives, shared through patient stories and testimonials, provide a unique and human perspective on the impact of medical interventions. In the case of Hyperbaric Oxygen Therapy (HBOT), these narratives offer glimpses into the lives of individuals who have embarked on a path of healing, often navigating challenges and celebrating successes along the way.

1. Wound Healing Triumphs:

Many patient stories centered around Hyperbaric Oxygen Therapy highlight remarkable successes in wound healing. Individuals dealing with chronic wounds, diabetic ulcers, or non-healing surgical wounds often share their experiences of how HBOT became a turning point in their healing journey.

One patient, for instance, may recount the frustration of a persistent diabetic foot ulcer that resisted conventional treatments. After undergoing a series of HBOT sessions, they witnessed accelerated healing, reduced infection risk, and improved overall wound management. These narratives underscore the transformative potential of HBOT in addressing complex wound healing challenges.

2. Overcoming the Aftermath of Radiation Therapy:

Patients who have undergone radiation therapy for cancer often face unique challenges related to radiation-induced tissue damage. HBOT emerges as a supportive modality in their stories, aiding in the recovery from conditions like osteoradionecrosis and soft tissue radiation injury.

In these narratives, individuals share how HBOT contributed to the restoration of bone health or alleviated the persistent pain and inflammation associated with radiation injury. The positive impact of HBOT on enhancing tissue repair and mitigating the long-term effects of radiation therapy becomes a recurring theme in these personal accounts.

3. Diving into Hope:

Decompression sickness, a condition afflicting divers due to rapid ascents, finds its way into patient stories of resilience. Divers who have experienced the bends share how HBOT became a vital part of their recovery process. These narratives often highlight the urgency of timely intervention and the effectiveness of HBOT in eliminating nitrogen bubbles, relieving symptoms, and preventing long-term complications.

From tales of recreational divers to professional underwater explorers, these stories weave a narrative of hope and recovery, emphasizing the importance of hyperbaric medicine in the context of diving-related emergencies.

4. Navigating Neurological Challenges:

The realm of neurological disorders introduces a spectrum of patient stories, each unique in its narrative and the challenges faced. Individuals recovering from strokes may recount their journey of rehabilitation, where HBOT played a role in enhancing neuroplasticity and supporting recovery.

Similarly, those grappling with traumatic brain injuries share their experiences of incorporating HBOT into their comprehensive treatment plans. The testimonials often highlight improvements in cognitive function, reduced post-concussion symptoms, and a renewed sense of hope in the face of challenging neurological conditions.

5. Pediatric Triumphs:

In the realm of pediatric applications, patient stories bring to light the resilience of children facing conditions like cerebral palsy or autism spectrum disorders. Parents and caregivers share how HBOT became a part of their child's therapeutic journey, contributing to improvements in motor skills, communication, and overall well-being.

These narratives not only showcase the impact of HBOT on the pediatric population but also emphasize the collaborative efforts of families, healthcare providers, and the children themselves in navigating the complexities of these conditions.

6. Beyond the Expected:

Some patient stories venture into unexpected territories, exploring the potential of HBOT in areas not traditionally associated with hyperbaric medicine. From accounts of improved mood and cognitive function in individuals with psychiatric conditions to narratives of enhanced athletic recovery and performance, these stories broaden the understanding of the diverse applications of HBOT.

These unconventional tales highlight the need for continued exploration and research to uncover the full spectrum of possibilities offered by HBOT in promoting health and well-being.

7. The Emotional Impact:

Beyond the physical outcomes, patient stories often delve into the emotional impact of undergoing HBOT. Individuals share feelings of hope, gratitude, and empowerment as they navigate their healing journeys. The supportive and collaborative nature of the hyperbaric team becomes a recurring theme, emphasizing the importance of a holistic approach to patient care.

8. Advocacy and Community Building:

Patient testimonials often extend beyond personal narratives to advocacy and community building. Individuals who have experienced the transformative effects of HBOT become ambassadors for awareness, sharing their stories to educate others about the therapy's potential benefits.

These advocates contribute to the creation of supportive communities where individuals facing similar health challenges can find encouragement, resources, and a sense of camaraderie. The power of shared experiences becomes a catalyst for building awareness and fostering a sense of connection among those exploring or undergoing HBOT.

In conclusion, patient stories and testimonials provide a powerful lens through which to view the impact of Hyperbaric Oxygen Therapy on individuals' lives. These narratives not only highlight the therapeutic potential of HBOT across a diverse range of conditions but also illuminate the resilience, hope, and sense of community that accompany the healing journey. As these stories continue to unfold, they contribute to a richer understanding of the human side of hyperbaric medicine, inspiring both those within the medical community and individuals seeking pathways to health and recovery.

CHAPTER NINE

Integrating HBOT into Clinical Practice

1. Collaborating with Healthcare Professionals:

The integration of Hyperbaric Oxygen Therapy (HBOT) into clinical practice requires a collaborative approach that involves healthcare professionals from various specialties. This multidisciplinary collaboration ensures comprehensive patient care, proper utilization of HBOT, and the exchange of knowledge among experts in different fields.

a. Involvement of Hyperbaric Medicine Physicians:

Hyperbaric medicine physicians play a central role in the integration of HBOT into clinical practice. These specialists are trained in hyperbaric medicine and are equipped to assess patients, determine the appropriateness of HBOT, and design individualized treatment plans. Collaborating with hyperbaric medicine physicians ensures that HBOT is administered with a thorough understanding of the patient's medical history, existing conditions, and potential contraindications.

b. Coordinating with Wound Care Specialists:

In cases where HBOT is utilized for wound healing, collaboration with wound care specialists is crucial. Wound care experts bring their expertise in assessing and managing complex wounds, and their collaboration with hyperbaric medicine physicians ensures a comprehensive approach to wound care. This collaborative effort aims to optimize the healing process and address the underlying factors contributing to chronic wounds.

c. Integration with Neurology and Neurosurgery:

When HBOT is considered for neurological conditions such as traumatic brain injury or stroke, collaboration with neurologists and neurosurgeons is essential. These specialists contribute their insights into the underlying neurological factors, ensuring that HBOT is integrated into a broader treatment plan aimed at maximizing neurological recovery.

d. Collaboration in Oncology:

In the context of cancer treatment support, collaboration with oncologists is vital. Integrating HBOT into cancer care requires a nuanced understanding of the patient's cancer history, ongoing treatments, and potential interactions with hyperbaric therapy. Oncologists play a key role in coordinating the overall cancer care plan while incorporating the supportive benefits of HBOT.

e. Coordinated Efforts in Pediatrics:

In pediatric applications of HBOT, collaboration extends to pediatricians, developmental specialists, and rehabilitation professionals. Coordinated efforts among these healthcare professionals ensure that HBOT is tailored to the unique needs of pediatric patients, addressing developmental considerations and optimizing outcomes for conditions such as cerebral palsy or autism spectrum disorders.

2. Establishing Hyperbaric Centers:

The establishment of dedicated hyperbaric centers is a pivotal step in integrating HBOT into clinical practice. These centers serve as specialized facilities equipped with hyperbaric chambers, trained staff, and the infrastructure needed to provide safe and effective HBOT services.

a. Design and Infrastructure:

Hyperbaric centers must be designed to meet safety standards and provide a comfortable environment for patients undergoing HBOT. This includes the installation of hyperbaric chambers, monitoring systems, and emergency equipment. The layout of the center should facilitate easy access for patients and healthcare providers, and attention to infection control measures is paramount.

b. Staff Training and Certification:

The successful integration of HBOT requires a team of trained professionals, including hyperbaric medicine physicians, nurses, and technicians. Staff members undergo specialized training in hyperbaric medicine, chamber operations, emergency procedures, and patient care. Certifications from relevant hyperbaric medicine organizations ensure that the staff is well-equipped to handle the unique challenges associated with hyperbaric chambers.

c. Patient Education and Support:

Establishing a hyperbaric center involves creating a patient-centered environment that emphasizes education and support. Patients must receive comprehensive information about the procedures, potential side effects, and expected outcomes of HBOT. Educational materials, pre-session briefings, and ongoing communication contribute to a positive and informed patient experience.

d. Collaborative Care Model:

Hyperbaric centers operate within a collaborative care model, fostering communication and coordination among various healthcare professionals. This model ensures that patients receive seamless care that addresses both the specific indications for HBOT and the broader context of their overall health.

e. Research and Quality Improvement Initiatives:

Leading hyperbaric centers often engage in research initiatives and quality improvement programs. Research contributes to the evolving understanding of HBOT's efficacy and expands its potential applications. Quality improvement initiatives focus on refining protocols, enhancing patient outcomes, and maintaining a high standard of care within the hyperbaric center.

f. Compliance with Regulatory Standards:

The establishment of hyperbaric centers involves adherence to regulatory standards set by healthcare authorities. Compliance ensures that the hyperbaric center meets safety, quality, and operational guidelines, providing assurance to both healthcare providers and patients.

g. Community Outreach and Awareness:

Hyperbaric centers actively engage in community outreach to raise awareness about the benefits of HBOT. Outreach efforts may include educational seminars, collaboration with referring physicians, and participation in health fairs. Building awareness contributes to a broader understanding of HBOT and its potential role in various medical conditions.

h. Continuous Improvement and Adaptation:

Successful hyperbaric centers embrace a culture of continuous improvement and adaptation. This involves staying updated on the latest research, incorporating technological advancements, and actively seeking feedback from patients and healthcare professionals. The ability to adapt to evolving healthcare landscapes ensures that hyperbaric centers remain at the forefront of patient-centered care.

In conclusion, the integration of Hyperbaric Oxygen Therapy into clinical practice involves collaborative efforts among healthcare professionals and the establishment of dedicated hyperbaric centers. Through multidisciplinary collaboration, coordinated care, and the creation of specialized facilities, HBOT becomes a seamlessly integrated component of patient treatment plans. The commitment to ongoing education, quality improvement, and community outreach ensures that the benefits of HBOT are maximized, contributing to enhanced patient outcomes and the advancement of hyperbaric medicine.

CHAPTER TEN

Future Directions of Hyperbaric Oxygen Therapy

1. Potential Innovations:

As Hyperbaric Oxygen Therapy (HBOT) continues to evolve, the future holds the promise of innovative advancements that may expand its applications, enhance therapeutic outcomes, and further refine treatment protocols. These potential innovations encompass technological, scientific, and clinical developments that could shape the future landscape of hyperbaric medicine.

a. Advanced Hyperbaric Chambers:

The development of more advanced hyperbaric chambers represents a potential innovation in HBOT. Future chambers may incorporate enhanced monitoring systems, customizable atmospheric conditions, and improved patient comfort features. Innovations in chamber design could contribute to a more tailored and efficient delivery of hyperbaric therapy.

b. Personalized Treatment Approaches:

Advancements in medical technology and our understanding of individualized patient responses may lead to personalized treatment approaches in HBOT. Tailoring hyperbaric protocols based on a patient's genetic profile, medical history, and specific health challenges could optimize therapeutic outcomes and minimize potential risks.

c. Integration with Regenerative Medicine:

The intersection of hyperbaric medicine and regenerative medicine presents exciting possibilities for the future. Research exploring how HBOT can synergize with regenerative therapies, such as stem cell treatments, may uncover novel approaches to tissue repair, organ regeneration, and overall health optimization.

d. Telemedicine Integration:

The integration of telemedicine into hyperbaric practice could enhance accessibility and monitoring of HBOT. Remote consultations, real-time monitoring of patients during sessions, and virtual follow-ups may become integral components of future hyperbaric care models, particularly for patients in remote locations.

e. Biomarker-Based Assessments:

Advancements in biomarker research may lead to the development of biomarker-based assessments for HBOT efficacy. Identifying specific markers that indicate a patient's response to hyperbaric therapy could guide treatment decisions and help clinicians tailor interventions based on objective physiological indicators.

f. Combination Therapies with Emerging Modalities:

The future may witness an exploration of combination therapies involving HBOT and emerging medical modalities. Collaborative approaches that integrate hyperbaric therapy with cutting-edge treatments, such as nanomedicine, targeted drug delivery, or immunotherapies, could synergistically enhance therapeutic outcomes across various medical conditions.

g. Artificial Intelligence in Treatment Optimization:

The integration of artificial intelligence (AI) into hyperbaric medicine may revolutionize treatment optimization. AI algorithms could analyze vast datasets, including patient responses, outcomes, and medical literature, to recommend personalized HBOT protocols. This could lead to more efficient and adaptive treatment plans, improving overall patient care.

2. Evolving Research Areas:

The future directions of Hyperbaric Oxygen Therapy are intricately linked with ongoing and evolving research areas. These research endeavors contribute to a deeper understanding of HBOT's mechanisms, refine its applications, and uncover new frontiers in medical science.

a. Neurological Disorders and Brain Health:

Continued exploration of HBOT's impact on neurological disorders and brain health remains a forefront research area. Investigating its potential in conditions like Alzheimer's disease, Parkinson's disease, and neurodegenerative disorders could unveil novel therapeutic avenues. Understanding how HBOT influences neuroplasticity, neuroinflammation, and cognitive function is key to advancing neurological applications.

b. Pediatric Neurology and Developmental Disorders:

Research in pediatric neurology and developmental disorders is likely to expand, exploring the nuanced applications of HBOT in conditions like cerebral palsy and autism spectrum disorders. Longitudinal studies assessing the impact of early intervention with HBOT on developmental trajectories and quality of life in pediatric populations could shape future therapeutic approaches.

c. Oncology Supportive Care:

The role of HBOT in oncology supportive care is a growing research area. Investigations into how hyperbaric therapy complements cancer treatments, reduces treatment-related side effects, and supports overall well-being may influence its integration into standard oncology care protocols.

d. Chronic Inflammatory Conditions:

Chronic inflammatory conditions, including autoimmune diseases, may become a focal point of research. Understanding how HBOT modulates inflammation and immune responses may open avenues for exploring its potential in managing conditions characterized by dysregulated immune activity.

e. Mental Health and Psychiatric Applications:

Research into the influence of HBOT on mental health and psychiatric conditions is an emerging area of interest. Exploring its impact on mood disorders, depression, anxiety, and post-traumatic stress disorder (PTSD) may shed light on the potential psychotherapeutic effects of hyperbaric therapy.

f. Metabolic and Cardiovascular Health:

The interplay between HBOT and metabolic or cardiovascular health is a research frontier with implications for conditions like diabetes, atherosclerosis, and vascular diseases. Investigating how HBOT influences metabolic pathways and vascular function may uncover therapeutic benefits in these health domains.

g. Global Collaborative Studies:

Future research efforts may involve large-scale, global collaborative studies pooling data from diverse populations.

Collaborative initiatives could facilitate the collection of robust evidence, allowing for more conclusive insights into the efficacy of HBOT across various medical conditions and patient demographics.

h. Long-Term Follow-up Studies:

Conducting long-term follow-up studies is crucial for understanding the sustained effects of HBOT. Research tracking patients over extended periods can provide insights into the durability of therapeutic outcomes, potential late effects, and the overall impact of hyperbaric interventions on long-term health and well-being.

i. Comparative Effectiveness Research:

Comparative effectiveness research may compare HBOT with other treatment modalities, offering a comprehensive understanding of its relative efficacy. Comparative studies could guide healthcare providers in selecting the most appropriate interventions for specific patient populations and conditions.

j. Health Economics and Cost-Effectiveness:

As HBOT becomes more integrated into clinical practice, research into health economics and cost-effectiveness is paramount. Evaluating the economic impact of HBOT in terms of healthcare utilization, resource allocation, and overall cost-benefit analysis will inform decision-making at both individual and institutional levels.

In conclusion, the future directions of Hyperbaric Oxygen Therapy hold exciting possibilities, from potential innovations in technology and treatment approaches to evolving research areas that explore the therapy's multifaceted applications. As scientific inquiry continues to advance, the integration of these innovations and research findings into clinical practice has the potential to elevate HBOT as a versatile and impactful therapeutic modality across diverse medical disciplines.

CONCLUSION

Summary of Key Points

In navigating the expansive realm of Hyperbaric Oxygen Therapy (HBOT), a multifaceted journey unfolds, marked by its historical roots, diverse applications, ongoing research endeavors, and the potential for innovative advancements. As we conclude this exploration, a synthesis of key points emerges, encapsulating the essence and significance of HBOT in modern medicine.

1. Historical Evolution:

The journey begins with a retrospective glance at the historical evolution of Hyperbaric Oxygen Therapy. From its inception as a treatment for decompression sickness in divers to its expansion into a versatile therapeutic modality, the historical trajectory underscores the adaptability and resilience of hyperbaric medicine.

2. Mechanism of Action and Physiological Effects:

At the heart of HBOT lies its unique mechanism of action, where increased atmospheric pressure and elevated oxygen levels converge to induce physiological responses. These responses, including enhanced oxygen delivery to tissues, anti-inflammatory effects, and stimulation of tissue repair mechanisms, form the foundation of its therapeutic impact.

3. Clinical Applications:

The diverse clinical applications of HBOT span a spectrum of medical conditions. From wound healing and decompression sickness to neurological disorders, cancer supportive care, and beyond, the versatility of HBOT is evident. Its integration into pediatric care further amplifies its potential impact, addressing conditions such as cerebral palsy and autism spectrum disorders.

4. Ongoing Research and Advances:

The landscape of Hyperbaric Oxygen Therapy is continually shaped by ongoing research initiatives and emerging therapeutic areas. Current studies explore the therapy's efficacy in traumatic brain injuries, chronic wounds, inflammatory bowel disease, cancer treatment support, and even psychiatric conditions. These research endeavors represent a dynamic field that propels hyperbaric medicine into new frontiers.

5. Safety and Side Effects:

Ensuring the safety of patients undergoing HBOT is paramount. Rigorous safety protocols, comprehensive patient screening, and vigilant monitoring during sessions mitigate potential risks. Understanding common side effects, such as barotrauma, oxygen toxicity, and temporary vision changes, allows healthcare providers to manage these effects effectively.

6. Patient Stories and Testimonials:

In the fabric of HBOT, patient stories and testimonials weave a narrative of hope, resilience, and healing. From triumphs in wound healing to overcoming the aftermath of radiation therapy and navigating neurological challenges, these stories provide a human perspective on the transformative power of HBOT. They also contribute to advocacy and community building, fostering awareness and support.

7. Integrating HBOT into Clinical Practice:

The integration of Hyperbaric Oxygen Therapy into clinical practice demands collaborative efforts among healthcare professionals and the establishment of specialized hyperbaric centers. Collaborating with hyperbaric medicine physicians, wound care specialists, neurologists, and oncologists ensures a comprehensive approach tailored to individual patient needs. Dedicated hyperbaric centers, equipped with advanced chambers, trained staff, and patient-centric infrastructure, serve as hubs for delivering safe and effective HBOT.

8. Future Directions:

The horizon of Hyperbaric Oxygen Therapy extends towards potential innovations and evolving research areas. Advanced hyperbaric chambers, personalized treatment approaches, integration with regenerative medicine, and the use of artificial intelligence signify potential innovations. Meanwhile, research areas spanning neurological disorders, paediatric applications, mental health, and oncology support indicate the dynamic future of hyperbaric medicine.

9. Conclusion and Forward Momentum:

In conclusion, Hyperbaric Oxygen Therapy stands at the intersection of tradition and innovation, weaving together historical roots with future possibilities. The therapy's multifaceted nature is evident in its ability to address a wide array of medical conditions while adapting to emerging research and technological advancements.

As we move forward, the momentum in hyperbaric medicine is driven by a commitment to patient-centered care, ongoing research, and a collaborative approach among healthcare professionals. The integration of HBOT into clinical practice is not merely a standalone intervention but a dynamic element within the evolving landscape of modern medicine.

The journey through the chapters of Hyperbaric Oxygen Therapy reveals not just a treatment modality but a tapestry of healing narratives, scientific exploration, and a commitment to advancing healthcare. Whether through the lens of historical milestones, physiological intricacies, clinical applications, or future horizons, HBOT emerges as a dynamic force contributing to the well-being of individuals across a spectrum of health challenges.

As healthcare providers, researchers, and advocates continue to navigate the realms of hyperbaric medicine, the essence lies in the stories of resilience, the pursuit of knowledge, and the shared goal of enhancing patient outcomes. Hyperbaric Oxygen Therapy, with its rich history and promising future, remains a testament to the enduring quest for healing and the potential for transformative advancements in the realm of medical science.

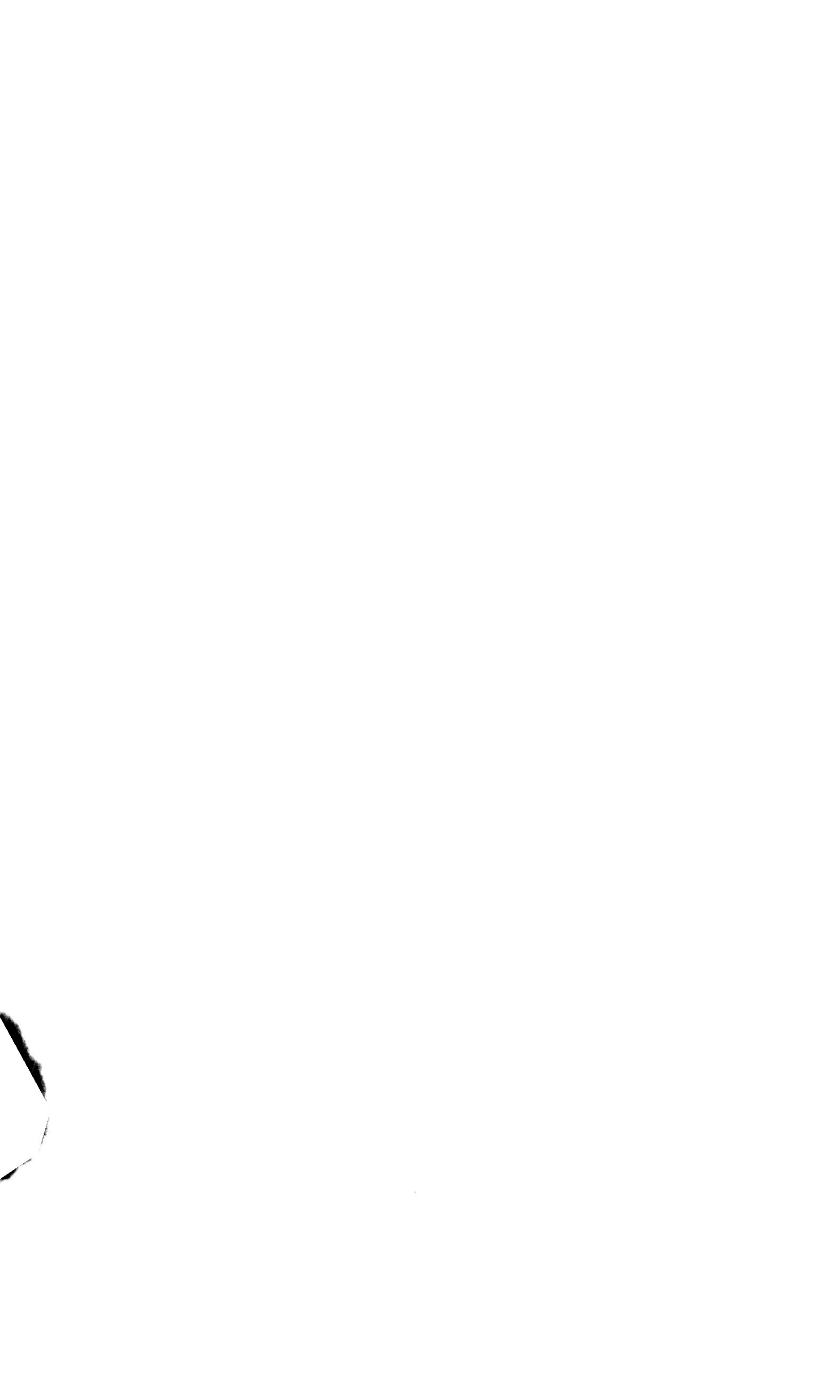